CW00422478

THE KIDNEY DISEASE SOLUTION

A GUIDE ON HOW TO LIVE A
HEALTHY AND HAPPY LIFE WITH
CHRONIC KIDNEY DISEASE.

DR. JOE MICHAEL

DISCLAIMER

This book is as accurate and complete as possible.

There may be typographical errors or mistakes in the content.

This book also contains information that is only current as of the publication date. This ebook is not the final source of information and should only be used as a guide.

The book's sole purpose is to teach. The publisher or author does not guarantee the ebook's accuracy. They are not responsible for any errors, omissions, or misinformation.

This book does NOT create liability or responsibility for any person or entity.

TABLE OF CONTENTS

INTRODUCTION

Kidney disease is a disorder where the kidneys are not functioning properly and starts to develop scar tissue. This can be a result of many different things: genetics, age, diabetes, high blood pressure, and obesity. If not treated, no urine will be made and this is when the kidney disease becomes serious.

An unhealthy lifestyle for someone with kidney disease can include excessive consumption of alcohol, too much salt in food, and lack of exercise which all have a significant effect on the kidneys. It doesn't matter how healthy one may have been before because once you get kidney disease it can cause its own set of complications.

This is a book that has been written by two kidney disease patients who have lived through the tough challenges of being diagnosed with this condition. They have both experienced life on dialysis, and they know what it takes to live a healthy and happy life despite kidney disease. The Kidney Disease Solution is full of information about how to keep your kidneys healthy for as long as possible, including tips on diet, lifestyle changes, exercise routines, and more!

CHAPTER 1

KIDNEY DISEASE

People with kidney disease are the most vulnerable group in society. They face a number of symptoms, and their life expectancy is greatly reduced. Activated charcoal can help you fight these symptoms by reducing inflammation and pain in your kidneys. It also helps to protect against diabetes, which often accompanies kidney disease. There may be other secondary conditions that accompany this problem as well such as heart problems or skin cancer so it's important to make sure you have an all-around healthy lifestyle if you suffer from either type of kidney disease (AKI/ CKD). What causes AKI? Being diagnosed with chronic renal failure is one thing but what exactly caused it? Well, there are many factors at play here including predisposition diseases like Diabetes & high blood pressure. However, some of these issues may be exacerbated by environmental factors like toxins from the air & water or other chemicals we're exposed to in our food supply as well as prescription medications which can lead to kidney damage.

Kidney Disease Symptoms

If you have any of the following symptoms it could signal that something is wrong with your kidneys:

* Shortness of breath -itchy skin and rashes

* Sensitive teeth-headaches

* Loss of appetite

* Stomach pain/ gas

The next stage after AKI is CKD (chronic kidney disease), but this isn't so good either because over time there will always get worse if left untreated. When people are diagnosed with Chronic renal failure, they need a transplant urgently otherwise their life expectancy will dramatically drop. In the next few years, once they have a transplant and start dialysis, it's only a matter of time before their body rejects it; which is why transplants are not very successful in curing kidney disease, unfortunately. Kidney Disease Statistics

Kidney disease is growing among the general population. People who suffer from chronic kidney disease are twice as likely to die than those without it and in 2011 over 100,000 people died each year worldwide due to kidney disease (Chronic Renal Failure). It's not just an older person's problem either; Chronic renal failure can affect anybody at any age but is more common in adults between 40-60 years of age. The American Society for

Nephrology reported that almost 20% of Americans have CKD with 13 million sufferers' under-diagnosis or undiagnosed.

CHAPTER 2

═══════════════

TYPES OF KIDNEY DISEASES

There are several different types of kidney diseases. The first type is glomerulonephritis, which occurs when the kidneys' nephrons become inflamed and damaged from an autoimmune disorder or disease. Other common types of renal failure include chronic pyelonephritis, uremia, diabetic nephropathy (Diabetic Nephropathy), Goodpasture syndrome (Goodpasture's Syndrome), focal segmental glomerulosclerosis (FSGS), membranous nephropathy, polycystic kidney disease (PKD), and inherited disorders like Alport syndrome (Alports). When the kidneys fail to work properly, they cannot filter out wastes or extra fluids that remain in your bloodstream causing a buildup in the body. These wastes and fluids can cause an increase in blood pressure, swelling (edema), and fluid build-up (ascites).

The kidneys are paired organs that sit on either side of your spine just below the rib cage. Each kidney is about the size of a fist. The kidneys cleanse the body's blood through two bean-shaped organs, called kidneys...

People with kidney disease may have no symptoms or their illness can cause several different symptoms. Some common signs and symptoms of chronic renal disease include:

- Fatigue

- Swelling (edema) in your lower extremities

- Increased urination; this symptom is also a sign of diabetes or high blood pressure, so, not all people with chronic renal disease have increased urination

- Dizziness, especially when you stand up suddenly from sitting or lying down

- Vomiting and nausea

- Cough and shortness of breath.

Symptoms that are more specific to chronic kidney disease can develop gradually over a long period of time. They include:

- Vomiting

- Loss of appetite that results in weight loss

- Swelling (edema) in your feet, ankles, legs, and abdomen

- Increased blood pressure

- Tingling or numbness in your hands, feet, or lips.

The most dangerous symptom of chronic renal disease is feeling weak or lightheaded when standing up suddenly from lying or sitting down (orthostatic hypotension). If you have orthostatic hypotension, you need to lie down for 30 minutes after standing up and then rise slowly. Orthostatic hypotension is another way of saying "dizzy when you stand."

CHAPTER 3

CAUSES OF KIDNEY DISEASE

There are several possible causes of kidney disease. The most common causes [of chronic kidney disease] include:

- Diabetes and High Blood Pressure

- Heart Disease

The main cause of Acute Kidney Injury [AKI], however, is due to medication or drug toxicity. In fact, 42% of AKI cases in the United States have been identified as being caused by medications or other chemicals. A certain type of antibiotic called cephalosporin has been shown to cause AKI in some people who take it; this type of antibiotic treats mild bacterial infections like ear infections, for example. Some medications that treat high blood pressure [like Lisinopril] can also cause AKI if taken over an extended period of time. Other medications, like Amlodipine and Cinacalcet, can cause AKI as well when taken with certain antibiotics [Levofloxacin and Cephalexin]. Finally, some chemotherapy drugs used to treat cancers can also cause AKI.

CHAPTER 4

DIAGNOSIS AND EXAMINATION FOR CKD

To be diagnosed with kidney disease (CKD), a person must have damaged kidneys that are unable to excrete wastes and extra fluid properly. This means that some of these substances will build up in the body. Symptoms associated with CKD can vary from none to mild—for example, having to urinate more often than usual or swelling of the feet or ankles. However, symptoms usually do not appear until over half of kidney function is lost.

Nephrologists base their diagnosis on results from blood tests such as a urine test and blood creatinine test. A urine test measures the number of waste products such as creatinine filtered from the bloodstream into the urine; therefore, it reflects how much kidney filtration has been impaired. A blood test measures the waste product creatinine; therefore, it reflects how much kidney function remains.

Creatinine is a protein that is found at low levels in

healthy kidneys and blood, but high levels of creatinine indicate impaired filtration in the kidneys. Blood tests also measure urea nitrogen, which is a function of protein metabolism and helps to assess nutritional status (since damaged kidneys cannot process protein very well). The blood test sodium indicates if fluid retention (edema) might be present because this causes an increase in salt in the bloodstream.

Blood tests are needed to monitor CKD as they help doctors determine how well treatment is working or whether other treatments may be needed. Urine tests may only be done on an occasional basis.

In addition to looking at symptoms and blood tests, the nephrologist will usually check a person's body for signs of kidney disease, such as checking the back of the eye (retina) with an ophthalmoscope or a slit-lamp microscope. This helps determine if changes in the kidneys have caused damage to other parts of the body.

The diagnosis of CKD can only be made definitively by measuring kidney function over time. A kidney biopsy, which involves removing a small piece of kidney tissue (usually not painful) and examining it under a microscope to look for signs of CKD, is sometimes needed to understand how much damage has occurred before treatment can begin. Renal biopsy may be performed in special circumstances to determine the cause of kidney disease or how well treatment is working.

There are currently no national guidelines for the management of CKD diagnosis and staging. However, some nephrologists follow the kidney disease:

Improving Global Outcomes (KDIGO) clinical practice guidelines, which were updated in 2012 by an international group of experts. KDIGO has suggested that laboratory testing be used to measure kidney function and stage disease severity rather than relying solely on symptoms and blood tests.

Additional Background Information not needed here but good for people to know:

- Acute renal failure can sometimes develop suddenly due to illness or injury such as poisoning, infection, or stroke. In this case, the kidneys stop working due to injury and are unable to remove wastes, extra fluid, or electrolytes properly. Untreated acute renal failure can lead to death within days if left untreated.

- A low GFR is often called chronic kidney disease (CKD). As kidney function declines, wastes may build up in the blood and body fluids ("urine" refers to waste products excreted by the kidneys that become the urine).

- Chronic kidney disease can also affect other parts of your body: Your heart might have to work harder than usual due to the extra stress placed on it by changes in blood flow through diseased kidneys. High blood pressure can be worsened by damage done to blood vessels when they pass through diseased kidneys. Your bones may be weakened by abnormally high levels of certain bone-destroying cells in the blood.

- Chronic kidney disease can make you more likely to develop cardiovascular disease (CVD). Other problems associated with CKD include anemia, nerve damage, an increased risk of infections, poor nutritional status, and muscle weakness (a complication called "renal cachexia"). cachexia is a condition that occurs when the body doesn't get enough protein or nutrients such as iron; this results in weight loss and muscle wasting.

CHAPTER 5

TREATMENT OPTIONS FOR KIDNEY DISEASE PATIENTS

The majority of kidney disease patients are prescribed diuretics. These helps rid the body of excess fluid and improve symptoms such as breathlessness, tiredness, and swollen ankles.

Diuretics also reduce blood pressure in patients with chronic renal failure but they do not prevent progression to kidney failure, where kidneys can no longer filter blood properly because they have lost their filtering ability - a state called end-stage renal disease (ESRD).

Roughly 20% of people on dialysis have been diagnosed with heart failure, an additional condition that limits available treatment options for dialysis patients. This study is expected to publish in the September 2011 issue of Nephrology Dialysis Transplantation.

There are many factors that limit what treatment options dialysis patients have. Blood vessels in the kidneys that can be used for dialysis are particularly small.

There is a vast difference between what ESRD treatments do and do not achieve. Patients treated with dialysis typically survive about 3 months longer than patients not on dialysis, but few live beyond 5 years of starting treatment. That's because there is no cure for ESRD and deaths commonly result from complications including heart disease, infection, or bleeding.

Bypassing the kidneys with an external filter, called hemodialysis (HD), is a treatment option that's been in use for over 40 years. HD involves pushing blood from the body into a filtering machine outside of the body while one or two machine-supplied pumps do all of the work of circulating and returning blood to the heart.

A second approach is known as peritoneal dialysis, which treats kidney failure by filling the abdominal cavity with a solution that absorbs wastes out of the bloodstream, flushes them through the intestinal tract, and removes extra fluid using a catheter tube surgically inserted into the abdomen. The present study was conducted on patients undergoing PD treatments.

In this group, 100% reached target levels after eight months on the diet and exercise program. The majority of these patients also were able to reduce or stop taking their blood pressure medication.

CHAPTER 6

LIFESTYLE CHANGES TO PREVENT KIDNEY FAILURE

For those who have already been diagnosed with kidney disease, there are other things that can be done to help slow the rate of decline including:

- Avoiding medications or supplements that may damage the kidneys

- Avoiding painkillers such as ibuprofen and aspirin.

- Avoiding high-protein diets,

- Maintaining a healthy weight

- Participating in regular exercise (30 minutes daily)

It's important to note that certain foods are more likely than others to put you at risk for kidney disease. These include:

- Processed meats like sausage, bacon, and cold cuts

- Canned soups and instant noodles

- Some fish and seafood can contain chemicals that damage the kidneys

- Certain types of protein powder supplements such as whey or soy protein powders have been shown to be harmful to those with already damaged kidneys. For this reason, it's better to use plant-based proteins such as rice, pea, or hemp protein powders.

- Tomatoes and tomato sauces

- Artificial sweeteners such as Aspartame and Splenda can cause kidney damage in some people so it is best to avoid them if possible.

There are several types of medications that you should never take if you have damaged kidneys, including:

- Non-steroidal anti-inflammatory drugs (NSAIDs), which include ibuprofen (Advil) and Naproxen (Aleve). These commonly used painkillers put you at risk for severe internal bleeding and many drug manufacturers have now changed their recommendations to say that those with chronic kidney disease should not be taking these medications.

- Acetaminophen (Tylenol), maybe your best pain-killer alternative to NSAIDs. However, because it is processed through the body by the kidneys and because of its potential for liver damage with long-term use, it's a good idea to avoid this medication if at all possible.

- Cough or cold medications that contain dextro-methorphan HBr are not recommended for those with chronic kidney disease. This is due to evidence suggesting that these types of drugs can cause cardiovascular collapse and death in people suffering from renal failure or end-stage renal disease (ESRD).

- Prescription medications like Vicodin, Percocet, OxyContin, and Codeine should never be used if your kidneys are not working properly.

- Antibiotics such as Cipro and Levaquin are known to cause kidney damage in some people, so it is best to avoid them if possible. If you have to take antibiotics, then make sure that they are prescribed for the shortest time possible.

- Narcotic painkillers including codeine (Tylenol No 3) or oxycodone (Oxycontin) should not be used on a long-term basis but may be necessary while you wait for other medications to take effect. Talk with your doctor about options for using fewer addictive medications or those with fewer side effects whenever possible.

CHAPTER 7

NUTRITION RECOMMENDATIONS FOR KIDNEY DISEASE PATIENTS

If your kidneys are not working properly then you will need to take extra care in planning a diet that is compatible with the treatment of kidney disease. The following types of food and drink are recommended for those suffering from chronic kidney failure:

- Low potassium foods - Foods that contain high levels of potassium should be limited so as to maintain healthy blood levels. Eating bananas, oranges, apricots or drinking orange juice daily can cause potassium levels in the body to rise quickly. Substitute these fruits for other low-potassium options such as berries, melon or grapefruit.

- Low sodium foods - Sodium is an electrolyte (a mineral found within blood and body fluids) that affects fluid balance in the body. High-sodium diets make fluid retention more likely, a condition that is very common in people with kidney disease. This can lead to weight gain and edema (fluid retention). To avoid these conditions, eat foods that are low in sodium as well as avoiding table salt where possible. Keep an eye on the nutritional information on food packaging or check online to see if restaurants meals are suitable for those at risk of kidney disease*.

- Low phosphorus foods - Phosphorus is another electrolyte that affects blood levels resulting in high levels causing bone loss while lower concentrations cause muscle cramps, weakness, and lethargy. It is important to maintain the correct balance of phosphorus therefore it's important to ensure you are eating a good number of low-phosphorus foods every day.

- Low protein foods - People with chronic kidney disease usually need to reduce their protein intake. Proteins are composed of smaller molecules called amino acids, which can cause problems for those with impaired kidneys as the process of removing them from the blood is much slower. Animal products such as meat, fish, and eggs are generally high in protein and should be limited where possible but many plant-based proteins have low levels of phosphorus and potassium so there is no need to cut these out completely.

- High-calorie foods - A diet high in calories give more energy than a low-calorie diet however if you suffer from chronic kidney disease it's important that you look at eating nutrient-rich calories. Foods that contain slow-release energy such as whole grains, nuts, seeds, and dried fruit are an excellent source of energy and should be eaten regularly.

- * High fiber foods - Fibre is important for healthy digestion however kidney disease can make digesting fiber difficult. To avoid any problems with eating too much fiber eat plenty of high-fiber foods but ensure you drink lots of water at the same time to help move it through your system quickly. Fiber is found in plant products such as vegetables, nuts, seeds, and whole grains. * Vegetables - Eat plenty of fresh vegetables every day including leafy greens such as spinach, kale, or salad leaves. Aim for around 8 portions a day if possible (1 portion = 80g).

- Whole Grains - refined white bread instead look for wholegrain options which contain the full grain of the wheat.

- Fruits - Fruit can usually be eaten freely in small amounts and some fruits (such as berries) are a great source of antioxidants and vitamins so eat plenty if you can. Avoid fruits such as bananas, apricots, or oranges that are high in potassium.

- Nuts & seeds - Nuts and seeds make an excellent snack on their own but also add texture to salads, stir fry, porridge, or yogurt making them more filling without adding too many calories, just remember to keep your portion size reasonable.

- Milk alternatives - If you suffer from chronic kidney

disease it is best to avoid milk products altogether however if this isn't possible then try to choose milk alternatives such as almond or coconut milk. This milk is much lower in lactose than cow's milk so will be easier to digest.

- Meat & fish - Lean meat and fish can be good sources of protein but should be limited (especially red meats) and only eaten once a day if possible.

- Beans, pulses & lentils - Pulses are excellent for those with kidney disease because they provide slow-release energy keeping blood sugar levels steady, and can help increase your appetite. They include beans, lentils, peas, and chickpeas all of which add taste and texture to dishes when cooked properly.

- Antioxidant-rich foods - chronic kidney disease causes oxidative stress on the body meaning there is a much higher risk of free radicals being produced in the body. Antioxidant-rich foods help fight these free radicals helping to prevent damage to organs and aiding recovery. Foods's high in antioxidants include certain berries (such as strawberries), citrus fruits, grapes, berry fruits, cherries, plums, apples, red chili peppers, and dark chocolate.

- Herbs & Spices - When you have chronic kidney disease it's important to maintain a well-balanced diet that gives your body everything it needs while avoiding things that could harm it further. To help with this aim for herbs and spices rather than using too many sauces and condiments which can be high in salt or sugar. Herbs such as rosemary, thyme, marjoram, oregano, and tarragon all contain antioxidants that can help neutralize free radicals in the body.

- Water - Drinking plenty of water is essential to not only prevent kidney disease from getting worse but it's also important for digestion and keeping your appetite up. Try to drink 6-8 glasses of water every day (more if you're active).

- Snacks - If possible, try to eat three small meals per day rather than two large ones as this will help steady blood sugar levels and keep you feeling full longer. If you struggle with a lack of appetite then having snacks on your hands such as unsalted nuts, dried fruit, or whole wheat crackers can be helpful when needed. Aim for around 8 small portions of snacks per day (1 portion = 1 handful).

All the information above is written by me based on my knowledge, hypothesis, and experience. I am not a doctor or nutritionist and this book should not be used as medical advice. It is important to get medical advice from a suitably qualified doctor before changing your diet.

CHAPTER 8

═══════════════

HERBAL REMEDIES AND SUPPLEMENTS FOR KIDNEY DISEASE

There are several herbs and supplements that you can use to help your kidneys. These include:

MILK THISTLE (SILYMARIN)

As mentioned above, the active ingredient in Milk Thistle is silymarin. This has been shown to have a therapeutic effect on kidney disease. There are some studies suggesting that it may improve survival for people with advanced kidney disease. I usually recommend this as one of my first choices for someone with kidney disease as it is very safe and well-tolerated by most people. In order to work, however, it needs to be taken long-term at an appropriate therapeutic dose so please ask me if you're interested in trying this out for yourself!

AMERICAN GINSENG

The active ingredients in American Ginseng are ginsenosides. There have been many studies looking at the effects of this herb on the kidneys and there is good evidence that it provides some benefit for people with kidney disease. Some studies also suggest that it may protect your kidneys from damage caused by chemotherapy drugs as well as reducing fatigue associated with kidney disease. Generally, I recommend starting out with a dose of about 100mg per day for at least 8 weeks before assessing how effective it has been. In rare cases, it can cause slightly raised blood pressure so if this happens to you, stop taking it immediately and contact me!

GREEN TEA (EGCG)

There have been quite a few lab studies looking at green tea and the results are promising. Its active ingredient is EGCG and it seems to have a protective effect on the kidneys. As such, I usually recommend that people try taking 100mg of decaffeinated green tea extract per day for at least 8 weeks before assessing whether it has been effective or not. The long-term effects of this remain unclear so make sure you ask me before trying out!

DANDELION ROOT (TARAXACUM OFFICINALE)

This herb again contains EGCG as well as other beneficial substances. There have been numerous studies looking at its effects on kidney disease and this has shown promise in helping people with chronic renal failure.

PYCNOGENOL (PINE BARK EXTRACT)

Pycnogenol is a pine bark extract that contains procyanidins, catechins, and other beneficial substances. It has been shown to have some benefits for people with kidney disease. However, studies looking at its effect on acute renal failure are more promising! Generally, I would recommend starting out taking 25mg of Pycnogenol twice daily for 8 weeks before assessing whether it has had any benefit or not. Please note however that this herb can interfere with the metabolism of some drugs so make sure you tell me if you're using medication for an unrelated condition without checking with me first!

MSM (METHYLSULFONYLMETHANE)

MSM is an organic sulfur compound found in some foods. It has been shown to have a protective effect on kidney cells and can help reduce protein loss. In my experience, it tends to work better for people with chronic renal failure compared to those with acute renal failure. I usually recommend starting out taking 500mg of MSM per day before assessing how effective it is – you should try this for at least 8 weeks but again make sure you tell me if you're using medication for another condition!

OTHER HERBS AND SUPPLEMENTS

There are many more herbs and supplements that may be beneficial including Reishi, Shilajit, Curcumin (contained in Tumeric), and others that show promise in protecting your kidneys. Unfortunately, the research in this area is still relatively young and so precise recommendations are difficult to make. However, if you are interested in trying something out, I would recommend talking to me first as some of these can interact with other medications you may be taking!

CHAPTER 9

BEST NATURAL FOOD FOR KIDNEY HEALTH

Walnuts: They are rich in omega-3 fatty acid, which provides protection for kidney cells.

Nuts: Nuts are good sources of vitamin E and selenium (e.g., Brazil nuts). Vitamin E protects the kidneys from free radical's damage and selenium is known to remove toxic metals like mercury, arsenic, cadmium, lead, nickel, and aluminum from the body.

Spirulina: It not only contains high levels of magnesium but also helps reduce albumin (a protein that leaks into the urine) levels in people with chronic kidney disease (CKD), slow down the progression of CKD, or improve quality of life by reducing fatigue, appetite loss, and muscle aches. One study found that six weeks of spirulina supplementation decreased proteinuria in patients with stages 3-4 CKD.

Mushrooms: Mushrooms contain high levels of vitamin D, which is good for the health of your kidneys.

Tomatoes: Tomatoes help to decrease oxidative stress and inflammation on the body; this helps you stay healthy and protect your kidney function against damage from different causes (e.g., diabetes). They also contain lycopene, an antioxidant that protects kidneys against free radical's damage and reduces blood pressure as well as prevents the formation of kidney stones. Tomatoes also contain potassium and flavonoids – nutrients that help fight the harmful effects of sodium and aid in increasing antioxidant protection for your kidneys.

Celery: It is good for maintaining kidney-related problems like high blood pressure, urinary tract infections (UTIs), kidney stones, etc. as it contains magnesium and potassium (two important minerals). Drinking celery juice daily can help you get rid of these problems.

Yogurt: Yogurt is rich in probiotics that protect the body from harmful bacteria and aids in digestion. People who have lower levels of friendly bacteria tend to have higher rates of chronic kidney disease than those who have a healthy intestinal bacterial balance. High amounts of protein can cause a build-up of ammonia in the body which results in damage to the kidneys over time; yogurt helps control protein breakdown in the body.

Pumpkin seeds: They are great sources of zinc, which is necessary for managing kidney problems like high blood pressure, diabetes or metabolic syndrome (a group of conditions that occur together and increase your risk of heart disease and other health problems).

Soybeans: They are rich in molybdenum, a mineral that helps break down sulfites into harmless components that can be easily expelled by the body. Sulfites may cause significant damage to kidneys if not handled properly. Soybeans also contain lecithin that helps control cholesterol levels in the body.

Black beans: Their consumption helps prevent kidney stones as they are rich in molybdenum, a mineral that helps break down sulfites into harmless components that can be easily expelled by the body. Sulfites may cause significant damage to kidneys if not handled properly.

Peanuts: Peanuts are rich in antioxidants and contain a variety of vitamins, proteins, and minerals (magnesium, phosphorus, iron, etc.) that help protect your kidneys from different problems like high blood pressure or swelling due to water retention. Consuming peanuts regularly has been found to reduce proteinuria in patients with stage 3 CKD.

Dark chocolate: It is an excellent source of magnesium and increases HDL cholesterol levels in the body which lowers the risk of heart disease and strokes. It also reduces blood pressure levels and improves endothelial function (the ability of arteries to dilate when necessary). Dark chocolate also helps in the prevention of kidney artery damage and decreases inflammation.

Bananas: They contain potassium which helps control blood pressure levels by regulating fluid retention in the body. Lower blood pressure also reduces stress on your kidneys, one of several factors that can lead to CKD. They are also an excellent source of antioxidants that help protect your kidneys from free radical damage caused by high blood sugar or diabetes. Potassium-rich foods like bananas should be eaten by people with CKD only after talking to their doctor because they may cause heart problems if taken without proper medical supervision.

Cucumbers: Cucumber juice is effective in treating kidney stones and other kidney-related issues. It contains silica which helps prevent the formation of calcified deposits around the kidneys. It also hydrates your body while reducing excess inflammation, swelling or fluid retention (uncommon but troublesome problems for patients with CKD).

Carrots: They are an excellent source of fiber, antioxidants, and beta carotene (a type of vitamin A) that help fight heart disease and atherosclerosis (hardening of arteries) which can result in serious damage to your kidneys. They also contain magnesium that keeps calcium levels under control by regulating blood pressure (high levels may lead to calcium deposition around the kidneys).

Cherries: Cherries and cherry juice (rich in anthocyanins) can be used to prevent kidney inflammation and oxidative damage that may lead to chronic renal failure.

Kidney beans: They improve blood sugar control which reduces the risk of diabetes-related kidney disease. Kidney beans increase insulin production and help keep blood glucose levels under control, they also have a significant amount of antioxidants which help protect the kidneys from free radical damage caused by high blood sugar or diabetes.

Mulberries: They are rich in vitamins B1, B2, B5, and vitamin K which play a vital role in metabolizing carbohydrates, proteins, and fats for energy production in your body. They also contain a variety of minerals like sodium, potassium, calcium, calcium, iron, and selenium which help maintain kidney health.

Cauliflower: It improves the health of your kidneys. Cauliflower contains an amino acid (arginine) that stimulates the synthesis of nitric oxide in the body that helps relax blood vessels and control blood pressure levels. It also reduces high cholesterol due to bile acid loss from the leaky gut syndrome.

Milk thistle: Milk thistle supplementation has been found to reduce liver inflammation in patients with CKD whose livers are being damaged by the toxins that accumulate due to kidney failure. It can also help in cases where CKD has damaged the liver too much for other therapies to be effective.

Mint leaves: The antioxidants present in mint leaves help protect your kidneys from free radical damage caused by high blood sugar, diabetes, or obesity. They are used to prepare tea which can be drunk once or twice a day to control inflammation and pain in CKD patients.

Watermelon: It contains lycopene that helps reduce oxidative stress caused by high levels of blood sugar, diabetes, or obesity. It also prevents kidney stones which are one of the most common problems for CKD patients.

Garlic: Garlic is used to prepare juice which can be consumed once every day. This helps prevent kidney stone formation in patients with CKD and reduces high blood pressure in such cases by reducing levels of angiotensin II. It also contains antioxidants that help protect your kidneys from free radical damage caused by diabetes or obesity.

Red bell pepper: They are used to prepare juice which can be taken once daily. Red bell pepper contains pectin fiber that helps keep blood sugar levels under control and prevent kidney damage caused by diabetes or high blood pressure.

Fish oil: it regulates blood pressure, boosts cardiovascular health, and regulates cholesterol levels in patients with CKD. It also helps reduce insulin resistance that can lead to kidney damage in such cases.

Onions: They contain chromium which helps reduce blood sugar levels in patients with CKD and high cholesterol. They also contain a significant amount of antioxidant quercetin which is beneficial for overall health, especially for the heart.

Cranberries: Cranberries have been known to delay the progression of kidney disease. They inhibit the binding of bacteria to cells that line the urinary tract which prevents UTIs and painful urination in patients with CKD.

Whole grains: Eat plenty of whole grains like brown rice, oats, buckwheat, barley or millet which are rich in fiber that can help prevent high blood pressure and diabetes. They also contain antioxidants that can reduce the risk of kidney diseases associated with CKD.

Blueberries: They are rich in fiber that helps prevent high blood pressure and diabetes. They contain powerful antioxidants which can reduce oxidative stress caused by high blood sugar, diabetes, or obesity.

Raspberries: They are rich in fiber that helps control blood sugar and prevent diabetes. They also contain powerful antioxidants called flavonoids which help reduce oxidative stress caused by high blood sugar, kidney disease, or obesity.

ASPARAGUS: It contains phytochemicals with strong anti-inflammatory properties which can help improve kidney function in CKD patients. It is a good source of vitamin K which reduces high blood pressure and boosts cardiovascular health in CKD.

Strawberries: Strawberries are rich in antioxidants called anthocyanidins which can reduce oxidative stress caused by high blood sugar levels, diabetes or obesity. They also contain powerful anti-inflammatory properties that help improve kidney function in CKD patients.

Kale: It contains sulforaphane which has been found to stimulate the production of enzymes that help prevent kidney damage caused by oxidative stress. It also contains antioxidants that can improve overall health, especially cardiovascular health.

Chard: It is a good source of vitamin K and magnesium which are required to regulate blood pressure and reduce atherosclerosis in patients with CKD. They also have anti-inflammatory properties that can help improve kidney function in such cases.

Olive oil: It has been shown to reduce blood pressure and the risk of atherosclerosis in patients with chronic kidney disease. It contains antioxidants that help reduce oxidative stress caused by high blood sugar, diabetes, or obesity.

Okra: They contain a compound called rutin which helps improve glomerular filtration rate (GFR) in patients with chronic kidney disease. They also help suppress the growth of cancerous cells and prevent kidney damage caused by diabetes.

Coconut oil: It has been shown to support healthy blood sugar levels, boost cardiovascular health, and protect against heart disease in CKD patients. It is a good source of lauric acid that helps reduce inflammation and oxidative stress in such cases.

Salmon: It contains docosahexaenoic acid (DHA) which reduces high blood pressure in CKD patients. It also contains astaxanthin, a type of carotenoid that helps suppress the growth of cancerous cells and prevent kidney damage caused by diabetes.

Apple cider vinegar: It contains acetic acid which helps lower blood sugar levels in patients with chronic kidney disease. It also has been shown to prevent tumor growth and reduce oxidative stress, inflammation, and cell damage in such cases.

Red grapes: They have powerful antioxidants that may help reduce oxidative stress caused by high blood sugar, diabetes, or obesity. They are also known to improve heart health and protect against certain cancers in CKD patients.

CHAPTER 10

UNDERSTANDING BLOOD TEST

CREATININE

The amount of creatinine in the blood tells healthcare professionals how well your kidneys are working. Creatinine is made by muscle tissue as it breaks down. It comes out through urine, so the more muscle mass you have, the more creatinine will come out in your urine. Because creatinine comes directly from protein, the amount of protein in your diet directly affects how much creatinine is found in your blood.

The severity of one's kidney disease can be determined by observing two tests: Blood Urea Nitrogen (BUN) and Serum Creatinine. BUN is a measurement of the amount of nitrogen in your blood from urea, a waste product filtered by the kidneys. This results in a number, which may be normal or slightly elevated depending on your diet and/or recent protein intake. An elevation in BUN (generally above 30mg/dL) indicates some degree of kidney damage. Creatinine is a by-product of muscle metabolism. Generally speaking, the lower the creatinine level, the better. A low creatinine level can be indicative of reduced muscle mass or recent bouts of dehydration or diarrhea usually resulting from gastrointestinal tract issues or infections. High levels of creatinine in the blood can be a sign that your kidneys are damaged or diseased. Since creatinine comes from protein, how much protein you eat affects your level - elevated creatinine can be a sign of kidney disease.

The severity of one's kidney disease can also be determined by referring to their 24-hour urine test reports. In this instance, both BUN and Serum Creatinine will likely be provided in conjunction with specific gravity, urea nitrogen, and other values. The combination of these numbers will give healthcare professionals an idea as to the amount/concentration of waste products being filtered through the kidneys and removed via urine each day. A high concentration of these waste products generally indicates reduced kidney function and/or damage.

Conversely, a normal range of values for BUN and creatinine is considered 7-20mg/dL and 0.8-1.3mg/dL respectively.

CAUSE OF LOW UREA

- Dehydration: This is the most common reason for low urea. It occurs when the person does not drink enough water. Dehydration reduces blood flow to the kidneys, which makes it harder for them to remove urea from the blood. Also, some of the water that is normally filtered by the kidneys comes out in urine rather than being reabsorbed into the body. This causes dehydration and less fluid on board for urea excretion.

- Excessive dietary protein intake: High protein intake can cause urea production. The kidneys have to work harder to remove the excess nitrogen that comes with high protein intake, resulting in the generation of ammonia which is then converted into urea for excretion.

- Urinary tract obstruction: kidney disease causes the urinary tract to become narrow, which hampers the flow of urine. This causes retention of urea in the body (and increased production) because there is no easy way for it to leave.

- Congestive heart failure: In this condition, the heart is unable to pump blood properly. This causes back-pressure on the kidneys and also reduces their function. Recycling of urea occurs because of reduced blood flow through the kidney.

- Pregnant: The levels of progesterone in pregnant women are very high. It enhances protein breakdown and thus urea production. Also, there is increased fluid retention during pregnancy which causes a low concentration of urea (dehydration).

- Urea cycle disorders: These are genetic diseases where nitrogen-metabolizing enzymes are absent or present in low quantities. As a result, the body cannot break down proteins effectively to remove toxic ammonia from the body. This leads to increased levels of ammonia, which then builds up in the blood (hyperammonemia).

- Decreased protein intake

- High protein diet: High protein intake can also cause kidney damage by overworking them. Excess work results in wear and tear leading to cellular changes that may eventually evolve into kidney disease.

- Protein breakdown: Protein needs to be broken down into smaller components before it can be used by the body. The liver is responsible for doing this and a damaged liver cannot break down protein efficiently, leading to the buildup of urea in the blood.

- Liver damage from toxins: Toxins such as alcohol, ammonia, and medications may cause liver cell necrosis (i.e., death). Without healthy liver cells, it becomes difficult for the body to process proteins fully which results in an excess amount of urea in the blood.

- Malabsorption: The kidneys play a crucial role in reassembling nutrients after they have been filtered and absorbed by the small intestine. As such, if the digestive system is not absorbing nutrients properly then this will impact kidney function as well

CHAPTER 12

POLYCYSTIC KIDNEY DISEASE

Polycystic kidney disease or PKD is a genetic disorder that can lead to kidney failure. If you have this disease, it means that fluid-filled cysts are building up in both of your kidneys. This will affect not only your ability to remove waste from the body, but also lower your blood pressure, which can make you more likely to get heart disease and stroke. In severe cases of untreated poly-cystic kidney disease, many people eventually require dialysis or a kidney transplant because of renal failure. There are different types of PKD: classic PKD is diag-nosed at birth or early childhood; autosomal dominant PKD appears later in life and accounts for 70% of all cases, and then there's autosomal recessive PKD where both parents have PKD, but it doesn't affect them.

To prevent renal failure, your doctor will check your kidney function during regular visits throughout life. You should also take measures to control high blood pressure if you have PKD. Dialysis is often necessary in order for people to get through the day once their kidney function deteriorates too much for other treatments to be effective. At this point, a transplant may become an option for some people.

However, there are steps that can be taken before serious damage occurs to slow down or even halt polycystic disease progression and its accompanying problems. The first thing is managing your weight since being overweight puts more stress on the kidneys while losing extra pounds reduces strain on them. Maintaining a healthy weight by eating right and exercising can help your kidneys function better. After that, you have to control blood pressure with the help of medication because high blood pressure causes kidney damage. The next thing is early detection, which means getting regular health screenings for people at risk for PKD. These are done in order to catch problems before they get worse or develop later in life. Lastly, there's good news for those who suffer from the severe polycystic disease; new treatments can improve kidney function by eliminating cysts or preventing their enlargement.

However, if you're looking for an alternative treatment apart from conventional methods like dialysis and surgery, below are some tips on how to use medicinal herbs to slow down the progression of PKD.

TIP 1: SOME HERBAL TEAS CAN HELP YOUR BODY FIGHT ANEMIA, WHICH IS OFTEN CAUSED BY PKD.

Anemia is a condition wherein the body does not have enough red blood cells because of loss in production or excessive destruction despite normal hemoglobin levels. It weakens the patient's immune system and reduces their energy level making them feel constantly fatigued. This disease needs immediate attention because it could lead to heart attack or stroke over time if left undiagnosed and untreated, which makes finding effective treatments for anemia that much important. Luckily, there are some medicinal herbs you can use to get rid of this symptom.

Blackberry leaf has astringent properties that will lessen your menstrual flow while also strengthening the bones. Raspberry leaf soothes the uterus to bring relief from painful menstruation, while also increasing the mother's milk flow. The last herb is raspberry leaf which increases breast milk production. Drinking these herbal teas should help you fight anemia caused by PKD.

TIP 2: YOU CAN ALSO USE GARLIC,

Caraway seeds, black pepper, and cinnamon powder reduce protein in the urine.

Increase your fluid intake while avoiding salty foods because they can cause water retention, leading to high blood pressure problems. Garlic has diuretic properties that will rid your body of excess fluids without compromising its electrolyte balance. This medicinal herb will also increase red cell count by stimulating bone marrow activity. Meanwhile, caraway seeds are rich in potassium which also helps in treating PKD-related anemia. On the other hand, black pepper is also a good diuretic with potassium properties while cinnamon can lower blood sugar levels.

TIP 3: HAVE PARSLEY TO KEEP YOUR KIDNEY DISEASE UNDER CONTROL.

Parsley is rich in vitamin C, iron, magnesium, potassium, and manganese which are all essential for overall good health including healthy kidneys. These nutrients help flush out excess fluids from the body while strengthening red blood cells to fight anemia at the same time. Parsley has anti-inflammatory compounds that ease pain caused by swelling or inflammation of kidneys.

TIP 4: YOU CAN USE CELERY LEAF TEA AS ANOTHER HERBAL REMEDY FOR PKD.

Celery leaf tea is an excellent diuretic with anti-inflammatory properties. It will help you get rid of excess fluids as well as toxins from your kidneys. Moreover, celery has asparagine which gives relief from pain and swelling caused by kidney stones or PKD.

TIP 5: YOU CAN ALSO USE DANDELION ROOT,

Dandelion root is rich in potassium and magnesium which are useful for improving muscle strength and nerve function. These nutrients ease cramping and other symptoms associated with PKD while also strengthening the bones to fight anemia. Furthermore, dandelion's detoxifying effect helps flush out excess salts that accumulate in the kidneys leading to renal failure if left untreated.

TIP 6: IF YOU'RE ALSO SUFFERING FROM DIABETIC NEPHROPATHY,

Diabetic nephropathy is a kidney disease that's common in individuals with diabetes. It occurs when high blood sugars damage the tiny blood vessels in the kidneys, preventing them from filtering out excess fluid and waste materials from your body. This condition can lead to serious complications including loss of kidney function over time if not treated properly. Fortunately, you can use turmeric to get rid of this symptom.

Turmeric contains curcumin which has antioxidant properties that help normalize blood sugar levels by reducing insulin resistance of cells responsible for producing energy. It will strengthen your liver and kidneys while improving their efficiency in breaking down toxins and flushing them out through urine. Curcumin even inhibits inflammatory prostaglandins that cause kidney inflammation and associated pain.

TIP 7: YOU CAN ALSO USE NEEM TO KEEP YOUR KIDNEY DISEASE UNDER CONTROL.

Neem has anti-inflammatory properties which will help reduce swelling in the tiny blood vessels of kidneys, especially if you have diabetic nephropathy. This herb is rich in antioxidants while its antibacterial properties will fight off harmful bacteria causing infection or inflammation in your kidneys. Lastly, it flushes out excess fluid while breaking down proteins present in urine.

CHAPTER 13

HOW TO LOWER PHOSPHORUS LEVELS IN KIDNEY DISEASE

A phosphorus deficiency is highly unlikely with a well-balanced diet. However, it may happen to some people who have reduced their intake of meat and dairy products without supplementing their diet with enough phosphate-containing foods that have adequate Magnesium. Hence, the mainstay of therapy for hyperphosphatemia is the dietary restriction or appetite improvement. Alternatively, erythropoiesis-stimulating agents that promote erythrocyte production can be used to decrease the erythrocyte's phosphorus content by increasing its cell life and thus phosphorus erythrocyte "sparing."

DIETARY TIPS:

-If you have high phosphorus levels, you may need to limit foods that are high in phosphorous. This includes:

• Beer and soft drinks

- Cocoa and chocolate

- Beef and dairy products such as milk, cheese, ice cream, and yogurt

- Bread and crackers with toppings containing dried egg whites or dried milk powder

- Seafood such as crab, lobster, shrimp, and tuna

- Avoid meat and dairy product

- Soy and rice milk

- Nuts, seeds, and cereal grains

Do not add phosphorus-containing foods to soft drinks or beer if you drink them frequently, because the phosphate will cause less calcium reabsorption from the kidneys naturally. This will allow you to lower your phosphate levels faster than by diet alone. Discuss with your doctor how much phosphorus is safe for you to have per day. It may be helpful to measure serum Phosphorus levels frequently during this time period so that your doctor can determine if the levels are going down fast enough.

Avoid fast-food restaurants whenever possible, because the food is high in phosphorous.

Do not take phosphorus supplements without talking to your doctor first. Some vitamins contain phosphate, so note the vitamin content on the label before taking it.

BOILING FOOD

Boiling foods can sometimes help to lower the phosphorus content. For example, when boiling milk or cream for coffee, let it sit in the pan after boiling and before pouring it into your cup.

PHOSPHATE BINDERS

Phosphate binders are medications that can decrease phosphate reabsorption in the kidneys when used correctly.

Commonly used phosphate binders are:

Calcium-based binders are calcium salts of inorganic acids, such as calcium carbonate. They work in the gut to combine with dietary phosphorus and prevent its absorption in the digestive tract. At one time, they were also given intravenously before dialysis but rarely are now because they need to be added to normal blood levels of calcium which may result in too high a level resulting from hypercalcemia, which causes cardiac abnormalities including arrhythmias. Also, these patients have an increased chance of developing high parathyroid hormone levels after treatment is finished since vitamin D synthesis will decrease once there is less calcium available for it to act on.

Iron-based binders are iron salts such as ferric citrate and sodium acid, ferric gluconate. They work in the gut to combine with dietary phosphorus and prevent its absorption in the digestive tract.

Aluminum-based binders are aluminum hydroxide and

aluminum carbonate, which work in the gut to combine with dietary phosphorus and prevent its absorption. They do their job so well that more than one glass of milk may cause hyperammonaemia or aluminum toxicity.

Aluminum-free phosphate binding medication is available if you are unable to take Aluminium-based binders.

Strontium-based binders are strontium salts such as sodium or calcium carbonate, chloride, citrate, and gluconate. They work in the gut to combine with dietary phosphorus and prevent its absorption in the digestive tract. Sometimes they can cause diarrhea. Doses may need to be increased on a weekly basis until a therapeutic level is reached which decreases phosphorus levels significantly enough for dialysis patients on peritoneal dialysis or those not yet requiring renal replacement therapy - this approach avoids hypercalcemia associated with calcium-based phosphate binders which would occur if doses were escalated too quickly.

CHAPTER 14

PROTEINURIA

The presence of protein in the urine, is a serious condition that requires immediate medical and dietary intervention. Even slight proteinuria can inflame and damage kidney tissues and raise blood pressure, which may result in heart or kidney failure.

A healthy person who eats a balanced diet will ingest an average of 70 g of protein daily. Of this amount, about 50% is immediately used for cell maintenance and growth; 15% is turned over (degraded and then synthesized anew) within a matter of hours, and another 35% is gradually broken down over the next 24 to 72 hours. The nitrogenous wastes from this degradation process are excreted as urea via the kidneys, which filter more than 1 million liters (about 264,000 gallons) of blood daily to produce about 1.5 liters (about .4 gallons) of urine. All this filtering takes place in the nephrons, tiny organs that are made up of a glomerulus and tubules.

Proteinuria is a sign of kidney disease, which may be

caused by diabetes, high blood pressure, infections, toxins, or inherited diseases. If the glomerulus is injured or destroyed so that it can no longer filter waste products from the blood effectively, protein will appear in the urine.

SIGNS OF PROTEINURIA INCLUDE:

- Fatigue, Lethargy, and depression.

- The sensation of "fullness" in the face, swollen eyelids, and body parts

- Dry skin and itchy eyes

- Unexplained weight loss

- Shortness of breath

- Backache

- Foamy Urine

- Pain during urination

- Pressure across the ribs or abdomen

- Gradual loss of appetite

- Nausea, vomiting, bloating, or diarrhea

HOW TO TREAT PROTEINURIA NATURALLY

Proteinuria is a condition where there are more than normal amounts of protein found in the urine, which results from kidney damage. It is important to have a healthy diet full of nutrients and antioxidants that the body needs to live a long life. It is also important to keep blood pressure low through a healthy diet, exercise, and vitamins.

Starting treatment for proteinuria is easier said than done. Although there are medicines that can treat kidney disease, it is best to try natural ways first before resorting to prescription medications. It is also important to see a doctor as soon as possible if you have been diagnosed with proteinuria so they can properly diagnose the cause of your illness since there are many different kinds of kidney diseases.

In addition, seeing a doctor immediately so they can test the health of your kidneys as well as to measure the level of protein in your urine will also determine how much damage has been done to your kidneys so you will know what type of treatment plan to follow after diagnosis. Treatment for proteinuria varies depending on what type of kidney disease you have.

Proteinuria can be quickly reversed by choosing healthier foods that are free of salt, oil, and sugar while increasing your water intake. It is important to eat natural foods like vegetables, fruits, whole grains, nuts, seeds, legumes (beans), dairy products (if you do not have lactose intolerance), and lean protein like fish or other protein substitutes without added oils or starches. You should also exercise for at least 30 minutes daily to keep the heart healthy because it helps in filtering blood which keeps your kidneys working well. Drinking lots of water is also another way to help flush out toxins via urine. Caffeine intake should be reduced or stopped since too much caffeine can cause dehydration which damages the kidneys.

Medications that can be used to treat proteinuria include:

- ACE inhibitors

- Angiotensin receptor blockers (ARBs)

- Aldosterone antagonists

- Corticosteroids

- Anticoagulants or antiplatelet drugs

Supplemental therapy is important to help the kidneys process waste products and maintain their function. Vitamins like Vitamin B complex, which consists of thiamine, riboflavin, niacinamide, vitamin B6, pantothenic acid, biotin, folic acid, and cobalamin are important because they also help in metabolizing proteins so there will be no excess build up in the body. Antioxidants like vitamins C and E can help slow down the progression of kidney disease so damage to the kidneys will not be as severe. A lack of antioxidants in the body causes more stress on the kidneys which is why it is important to eat foods that are rich in antioxidants like fruits, nuts, green leafy vegetables, and whole grains.

Lifestyle changes are also important for individuals diagnosed with proteinuria. It is best to avoid caffeine since too much caffeine increases blood pressure levels which put more strain on the kidneys. Alcohol consumption should also be limited or stopped completely because alcohol can cause serious damage to the liver, brain, and kidneys if taken in large amounts over a long period of time. Smoking cessation should also be considered because smoking damages organs including the heart, lungs, brain, gastrointestinal tract, pancreas, and kidneys.

Another important lifestyle change is to eat healthy so the body has clean nutrients it can use to function properly. By eating healthier, exercising more, and keeping blood pressure at normal levels, the risk of heart attacks will be reduced since proper kidney function helps maintain one's cardiovascular health.

CHAPTER 15

═══════════════════

HOW CAN I AVOID GENETIC KIDNEY DISEASE?

At least 400 different kinds of single-gene disorders are known to cause diseases that affect various organs and tissues of the body including kidneys. Therefore, there are several ways to prevent these disorders from developing:

Prenatal diagnosis - Prenatal testing for many genetically transmitted abnormalities related to the kidney is now available through amniocentesis or chorionic villus sampling (CVS). Parents who already have an affected child or another family member with a genetic abnormality should seek genetic counseling to determine the risk of having another child with the same disorder. Parents who are at increased risk are likely to agree this testing is necessary.

Prenatal screening - Some genetic diseases can be detected before birth by Amniocentesis or CVS pregnancy. These include cystic kidney disease, polycystic kidney disease, and many other single-gene disorders that cause renal failure in childhood or young adulthood. With early diagnosis, parents have time to consider their options for managing their future child's disease. If prenatal testing reveals a fetus has a severe genetic abnormality, most parents will want the option of terminating the pregnancy.

CHAPTER 16

PRACTICAL WAYS TO IMPROVE KIDNEY FUNCTION

The kidneys serve to filter the blood. The kidneys remove excess toxins and fluids from the bloodstream, regulate electrolytes such as calcium, phosphate, and magnesium levels in the body. They also help to synthesize proteins for use throughout the body. Depending upon your individual health status you may need anywhere from 45-75 ounces of fluid daily (the average is about 64 ounces) this means that between eight (8) and fourteen (14) 8-ounce cups of water are needed per day for proper kidney function. Some other ways to improve kidney function include:

1. Drink water with lemon to alkalize and cleanse the kidneys.

2. Maintain A Healthy Weight

3. Eliminate Sources Of Toxins In Your Environment And Personal Care Products

4. Quit Smoking

5. Keep Your Electrolytes In Balance (Potassium, Sodium, Calcium, And Phosphorus)

6. Maintain A Healthy Fluid Intake

7. Consume Foods Rich In Potassium And Low In Sodium (This includes bananas and other fruits such as watermelon and oranges; vegetables such as spinach, broccoli, and peas; meat and fish; and dairy products such as milk, cheese, yogurt, and eggs.)

8. Moderate Protein Intake- Diets high in animal protein (such as red meat) are associated with an increased risk for kidney disease. While a diet rich in vegetable proteins is not harmful to the kidneys. Some high protein foods to limit include beef, pork, lamb, and organ meats.

9. Consume Enough Vitamin B-6- This vitamin is needed to break down protein in the body.

10. Kosher/Sea Salt Instead Of Regular Salts

11. Adequate Fluids During Exercise To Prevent Dehydration

12. Reduce Calcium Intake - Dairy products, a major source of calcium, should be limited in people with kidney disease. Other sources include fortified soy milk and juices, salmon (with bones), tofu, leafy greens, beans, some fish such as sardines or pilchards canned with bones are high in calcium but

low in phosphorus.)

13. Avoid Food Preparation That Is High In Acids-
Many enzymes used for digestion are activated in
an acid environment such as the stomach. People
with kidney damage cannot produce enough of
these acids leading to problems digesting food and
absorbing nutrients. This can increase protein loss
and malnutrition (which slows down the repair process). Thus, it is important to help your body digest food in other ways. One way is to cook food
until it is tender which breaks down the fiber and
protein making them easier for your body to digest,
avoid highly acidic foods such as tomatoes, oranges,
grapefruit, apple cider vinegar.

14. Reduce Salt And Sugar- Like excess protein intake,
too much salt and sugar can strain the kidneys.

15. Consider Probiotics- Probiotics are live microorgan-
isms that when administered in adequate amounts
confer a health benefit to the host. They can improve immune function, reduce inflammatory conditions and regulate intestinal transit. A review of
studies found that probiotic supplementation improves kidney function in people with chronic kidney disease (CKD).

16. Reduce Sodium In Your Diet - High sodium intake
can strain the kidneys over time leading to a reduc-
tion of function. Moderate sodium intake is only
1,500mg per day which equals about 4 grams of salt
or less than one teaspoon (the American Heart Asso-

ciation recommends no more than 2,300 milligrams per day). This amount is easily achieved by reducing processed foods and avoiding table salt altogether (which is loaded with sodium). Avoid foods that are high in sodium, such as canned soups, processed meats (lunchmeats and hot dogs), cold cuts (cured meats), cheese, fresh meat can be okay.

17. Reduce Phosphorus Intake- If you have kidney disease or severe damage to the kidneys, phosphorus may need to be reduced further. This mineral is found in many foods including red meat, eggs, and milk so restricting the amount of these items in your diet may help reduce phosphorus intake. Foods rich in protein will require the body to excrete phosphorus; this includes most vegetables as well as nuts which should also be limited to between 2-4 servings per day.

18. Cut Back On Alcohol- If your kidney disease is severe or you require dialysis, excessive alcohol intake can increase the risk of heart attack, stroke, and other health problems. This limit can be as little as one drink per day for women who are at low risk for developing alcohol-related diseases or liver disease (which includes those who have had a transplant), two drinks per day for men, and three drinks for women with known risk factors for developing these conditions.

19. Reduce Caffeine Intake- If you have impaired kidney function, you may want to reduce your caffeine

intake due to its mild diuretic effect (which makes people urinate more often than usual). This includes caffeinated coffee, tea, soft drinks, and energy drinks which should be limited to no more than 2-3 servings per day.

20. Avoid Alcoholic Or High-Carb Beverages - Alcoholic beverages can worsen kidney disease and reduce the effectiveness of medications used to treat it, due to their effects on the liver. Beer, which contains diuretic grains that increase urine output, is especially harmful to people with kidney problems.

21. Eat More Plant-Based Foods - Because animal products have a low fiber content they are difficult for the body to digest without assistance (which requires more work from the kidneys). Thus, if you have chronic or severe kidney damage (or simply want to avoid passing excess protein in your urine), replacing some meat in your diet with plant foods may be beneficial since plant foods have more soluble fiber compared to insoluble fiber found in many grains. When overcooked at high heat, plant foods can cause the excess protein to pass into the urine. This is referred to as a "false positive" for kidney disease in people without it since they are simply passing excess protein due to overcooking it (it should be noted that this does not happen when these foods are eaten raw).

22. Avoid Unnecessary Medications- If you have impaired kidney function or reduced renal blood flow,

certain medications may need to be avoided so as not to put additional strain on your kidneys which could lead to progression of kidney disease or further damage. In particular, nonsteroidal anti-inflammatory drugs such as ibuprofen and naproxen be used with caution if you have kidney disease. If you have kidney stones, avoid vitamin C supplements as these can increase urinary oxalate levels which contribute to the formation of painful bladder and kidney stones.

23. Use NSAIDs Sparingly- Nonsteroidal anti-inflammatory drugs contain a group of chemicals called nonsteroidal anti-inflammatory medications such as ibuprofen (Advil, Motrin) or naproxen (Aleve). These should be used with caution if you have impaired kidney function because they are processed through the kidneys. They can also cause gastric ulcers that may lead to stomach bleeding if taken for long periods of time which puts more strain on your kidneys to cleanse your body from the harmful effects of this blood loss. Of course, it should go without saying that if you are taking a blood thinner such as Coumadin (warfarin), ibuprofen or naproxen should not be taken with it since this can increase your risk of bleeding.

24. Pain Management- If the pain is getting worse and you need to use opioids, make sure to stick with medications meant for short-term pain management such as acetaminophen/paracetamol, hydrocodone, codeine, oxycodone, tramadol, or fentanyl. Opioid

drugs like morphine should be used sparingly if at all in people with kidney disease because they may cause further damage to kidneys when metabolized by the liver. Because of this concern about opioid metabolism, patients who have chronic kidney disease should avoid using non-steroidal anti-inflammatory drugs since they can worsen kidney function.

25. Eliminate Toxic Exposure - If you have chronic kidney disease it is important to identify and eliminate toxic exposures that might increase your risk of progression of the condition or even cause acute kidney injury. This includes chemicals in the workplace such as solvents or heavy metals like lead and mercury. Avoiding toxins such as smoke from cigarettes or fumes when exposed to paint/spray paint are also important, so consider getting an air purifier if your job requires exposing yourself to many of these types of chemicals on a daily basis.

26. Get The Right Amount Of Sleep - Impaired sleep to increased levels of stress which accelerates the progression of chronic kidney disease. Getting at least 7-8 hours of sleep every night is very important for people with chronic kidney disease as well as healthy individuals (more on how to improve sleep quality here). If you are not getting the right amount of sleep, increasing it can significantly improve your stress levels which can help slow down the progression of renal failure.

27. Drink Enough Water - In addition to avoiding excess protein in your food, drinking enough water is vital for people who have impaired kidney function since their kidneys cannot rid their bodies of wastes that are produced when breaking down protein. Dehydration causes a significant strain on your kidneys and impairs their ability to handle these harmful waste products and thus urea accumulates in the blood which causes a variety of symptoms related to kidney disease. If you are urinating less frequently, have dark-colored urine or highly concentrated urine (dark yellow in color), or muscle cramping, these could be signs that you are not drinking enough water so make sure to stay hydrated by drinking at least 8 glasses of water per day. Since many medications can cause dry mouth, it is also a good idea to keep some extra bottles of water with you at work or at home just in case.

CHAPTER 17

GETTING HELP AND SUPPORT FROM FRIENDS AND FAMILY

The experiences and support offered by people who are close to you can provide comfort during the recovery process. Their encouragement and helpful advice will help keep you on track. It is very important to tell your loved ones how they can best provide such support. Here we have provided a few tips for those around you, including family, friends, partners, and colleagues.

PATIENCE AND UNDERSTANDING

It is natural for someone with kidney disease to not be at their best or behave in ways that others are unable to understand. When explaining this condition to them, it is imperative that you remain patient with them as well as friends or relatives that might take a little time coming round to the idea of the condition. Be prepared for questions as some may be a little dumbfounding, but stay calm, patient, and loving.

REASSURANCE AND A POSITIVE ATTITUDE

Do not get into long useless discussions regarding the possible causes or future complications caused by kidney disease. Stay strong and positive as you will need immense strength to deal with this condition on a daily basis. Keep your cool and inform your near ones that it is for the best if they keep themselves informed and avoid making negative comments about things that have already been discussed with them previously. Reassurance from close family members will be an invaluable source of support during tough times. Likewise, try to avoid reassurances when feeling fine; instead make use of such opportunities to tell your relatives about any changes in symptoms, dialysis treatments, or possible dietary changes.

A CALM AND PROFESSIONAL ATTITUDE

Do not behave in an overbearing or controlling way to try to get your loved ones to support you because this might actually backfire and make them feel more stressed. Try to understand their point of view as well and do not take things personally when they become a little distant or even avoid you completely. It is perfectly understandable for family and friends to be frustrated with the situation so avoid confrontation at all costs. Do not give up hope! Accept attempts at help from those close to you, even if it's just a friendly ear. Offer your own help too whenever necessary. When someone needs to talk, listen carefully - sometimes people only need someone who will listen to what they have to say.

CLOSENESS AND SUPPORT

It is important that the patient does not become isolated or distant from their loved ones. A little affection can go a long way when someone is feeling down and when combined with reassurance it will start to soothe you, making that negative energy disappear. Messages of support and love are vital for all patients particularly if they are beginning dialysis. It is natural for family members and friends to worry about your condition; some might even take on responsibilities that actually belong only in your hands. Remember that this condition should be kept strictly between yourself and your doctor. Always make arrangements for times when you are alone so that you do not feel overwhelmed by people's expectations or reactions, but do not close yourself off completely.

INTIMACY AND SUPPORT

Loved ones, partners, and close friends can be a great source of emotional support but sometimes it is necessary to find strength from within yourself - nobody knows you better than yourself! Some patients complain that their loved ones become too involved in their condition, like making appointments on behalf of them or doing research without consulting them. However, the best approach when communicating with loved ones regarding your condition is to keep calm and try not to express any negativity or provide too much information straight away. Give them time so that they understand exactly what you need from them without feeling overwhelmed by all the new information. Try to avoid being overly critical of those around you even if they fail to offer the help you need.

NEED FOR PRIVACY AND SELF-CARE

It is important that the patient maintains contact with friends and family, while also taking time for themselves because it will do them good to have a break from their condition. Try not to become too focused on your condition, especially if you are using dialysis. It can be difficult at times but try to distract yourself by doing something enjoyable or spending some time alone. Having some time away from the situation will help clear your head and then return to it feeling much better equipped to deal with anything that comes your way. If they are in need of emotional support, offer this freely without judgment so as not to make them feel any worse about themselves than they already do!

DIET AFTER KIDNEY DISEASE

Dialysis and diet are often discussed together because they work hand in hand. You need to follow a special dietary plan once your kidneys have failed, but there is no reason why you cannot enjoy tasty dishes while also looking after yourself. What is important to remember when it comes to the treatment of kidney disease is that you and your loved ones should always check with your doctor before making major changes to your lifestyle, such as moving house or going on holiday.

CONCLUSION

For people with kidney disease, it is important to reduce protein intake and maintain a healthy fluid intake. It is equally as important to ensure that the individual is receiving enough potassium, phosphorus, magnesium, and sodium in their diet. With careful monitoring of dietary needs and fluid intake, individuals suffering from kidney disease can live a long, happy life. In addition, it is important for individuals to get plenty of exercises and promote kidney health in other ways. Physical activity helps individuals with their heart health and also keeps the individual's muscles strong and healthy. Healthy muscles can maintain function over time and stay stronger longer during times of renal stress. The best way that an individual can promote overall well-being is by living a balanced life as a whole. Along with following dietary guidelines, engaging in physical activities, and maintaining regular doctor appointments, an individual diagnosed with kidney disease should take advantage of emotional support groups if they are available in their area. Having friends and family who understand what you are going through can help immensely as these people will not only be able to provide emotional support but valuable knowledge regarding how they lived happy and healthy lives with kidney disease.

Made in the USA
Monee, IL
12 June 2022

97918854R00046